I0500773

By Cindy Wright

Acupuncture

*Holistic Therapies and
Alternative Health
Book 1*

Acupuncture
Cindy Wright

Also by Cindy Wright
Non-Fiction

The Popular Seaside Places of the United
Kingdom
Worlds of Ice
Part of Your World
Addition Package
The Dark Traveller
Christmas Magic for Children
The Different Ways of Celebrating Easter
Aerobics: A Guide to Keeping Your Heart and
Body Healthy
When Considering a Cat (Loving Your Cat 1)
A Journey through the Histories of the
Provinces of the Republic of Ireland

Candles (*Holistic Therapies and Alternative
Health Book 3*

Fiction

The Magic of Folly Meadow (Suzie's
Adventures of the spirit World 1)
Seal Island Adventure (Island Adventures 1)

Acupuncture: Its Genesis

The beginning of acupuncture hails back to about 2000 years ago in China. The term acupuncture may come from the Chinese, but it actually derives from the Latin words "acus" and "pungere". "Acus" means needle in English and "pungere" is referred to as prick.

Acupuncture has evolved in a variety of forms. There are techniques that do not use needles, but instead they use ultrasounds, vibrating objects and practitioner's fingers.

Looking back to its origin, acupuncture made its way into the realm of medicine when it was initially discussed in an ancient Chinese medical text, titled "Huang Di Nei Jing," in English, "The Yellow Emperor's Classic of Internal Medicine".

However, some archaeologists revealed that acupuncture was introduced even before the Chinese when a 5,000 year old mummy was unearthed in the Alps with acupuncture points in its body. Nevertheless, no text or history books could prove this sceptic anecdote; thus, the origins of acupuncture go back to China with regard to acupuncture's ancient practice.

The knowledge of this practice progressed in Japan in the 6th century. Then in the 17th century, a man formulated a painless procedure for patients by developing an insertion tube. It was a small cylindrical tube where a needle was inserted. The name of the man was Waichi Suyiyama. Thanks to him, some individuals in the practice began using his invention and continue to do so today.

The practice of acupuncture arrived in the US in the early 80's when the *National Commission for Acupuncture and Oriental Medicine* was established. Upon the establishment of the regulatory board, some schools were opened, inviting those who desired to be a professional and licensed acupuncturist. In spite of this progress, some people do not believe in the positive effects of acupuncture as an alternative form of medication. These people remained unconvinced until 1995 when the needles utilised for acupuncture were considered as a medical instrument by the *US Food and Drug Administration.* Because of the classification given by the government, the public became assured that the practice is effective and safe.

To further assure the effectiveness of acupuncture, the National Institute of Health or NIH affirmed the efficacy of this technique in treating many health conditions. Treatment includes disorders and maladies in the person's nose, ears, eyes, throat and bodily systems like muscular, nervous, gastrointestinal and respiratory. The good thing is, acupuncture has lesser side effects compared to conventional drugs that are promoted and sold by companies in the pharmaceutical industry.

NHI recommended that US companies should provide full coverage on definite conditions and make acupuncture available to the public. For those who will not qualify, partial coverage may be available, something that needs to be looked up in your coverage plan. However, there is a need to accumulate more resources or studies to prove the effect of the technique on other health related problems. Some health related disorders include autism, addictions, migraines, persistent lower back pain and osteoarthritis of the knee.

The needle technique can be traced to the history of acupuncture and is still the same method used today. Though there are a variety of forms developed as the years have gone by, one thing is definite, it is still effective. For more information on the effectiveness of the technique, visit a specialist on this field that is well-trained and qualified to treat your body's condition.

A Quick-Start Guide to Acupuncture

The principle of acupuncture is the use of needles to adjust or regulate functions of the body towards their optimum level. Practitioners of ancient Chinese and modern Western medicine utilise this practice to ease the pain experienced by those who suffer from chronic diseases. Relatively, using these needles is harmless; it is a positive strategy of treating pain, improving health and optimising a person's well-being. To know more about the procedure performed in the practice of acupuncture and its benefits, continue reading the information below.

Procedure for Needle Puncture

Today, two broad categories are practiced in acupuncture, the traditional Chinese medicine (TCM) and medical acupuncture. These two categories possess distinct intrinsic worth. Primarily, the choice to opt to either of the two categories depends on the individual and their thoughts on the practice, less on the technique performed.

Practitioners performing TCM stick to the concept of Qi or energy flow and the meridians where they pass through. Traditional Chinese Medicine utilises longer needles and introduces them deeper into the body to get in touch with the acupuncture points. Although, there are only a few bits of evidence that prove the existence of energy channels. As claimed by modern science, this technique has been very effective for thousands of years.

On the other hand, practitioners of medical acupuncture gained their learning from western medical schools. They apply needles based on anatomic data, not on the traditional points of the practice. Shorter needles are used by modern western practitioners who perform shallow insertions. They only use a few needles and allow them to be inserted for a short period of time. Those who adhere with TCM will say the western practice is a watered-down adaptation of the real technique. Apparently, plenty of patients stated that they experienced great relief after the application of this method.

Conditions for Puncture Application

There is a long list of ailments or maladies where this technique can be applied as a treatment. Ailments which can be treated by acupuncture include asthma, constipation, anxiety, weight loss and many others. In the realm of TCM, practitioners believe any health condition a person is suffering from is due to the disparity in the Qi flow, thus, needle therapy is best applied. However, controlling pain is still the most common ailment they treat.

Of all the indications for this technique, the control of pain is generally the most well researched ailment. When acupuncture is used as a treatment in ailments like migraines, arthritis, premenstrual syndrome, neuralgia and carpal tunnel syndrome, there are certain beneficial effects encountered by most patients. The gate-control theory of pain is the principle behind the effectiveness of the technique which is based on medical research and other studies. The theory states that through the needle, nerves can be stimulated to block 'trigger' impulses of pain.

Expected Puncture Session Result

On top of an existing medical treatment, acupuncture can still be utilised Patients should not stop taking their medication or neglect medical instructions related to needle puncture. Once a patient undergoes a needle puncture treatment, the doctor in charge of the patient's primary care will make an assessment in relation to lessening the person's dependence on other therapies.

Patients who undergo acupuncture therapy have to wait for a few weeks or even months to finish the treatment. Generally, the duration relies on the intricacies of a certain medical condition, better yet, various results can be expected. It is very important to have an honest conversation with the acupuncturist about the results to look ahead to, and the time frame of the course. Oftentimes, patients will experience beneficial effects after 3-4 sessions. Thus, it would be better to be informed time after time of the reasons for specific conditions which may get worse before improvements can be attained.

Traditional techniques are widely accepted in modern medicine so long as the results of the practice are proven to be effective. Time and again, acupuncture has proven its significance. With the modern guidelines implemented for this practice, it proves that it is reproducible, safe and effective to provide healing to millions of people who need relief in times of pain or when an ailment occurs.

Understanding Acupuncture

Acupuncture is defined as a holistic form of health care that is utilised to inhibit and cure some diseases as well as help the patient to achieve relief from pain and anesthetisation from certain surgeries. According to research, this practice was introduced in China and has been used for more than 5,000 years.

The earliest text that lead to the familiarisation of acupuncture was found in the book titled, "The Yellow Emperor's Classic of Internal Medicine" or known in Chinese as "Nei Jing". The text of this book was written by its proponents during 200 BC. Practitioners at those times used needles made out of stone, herbs and moxibustion in treating patients. Today, the needles used are made from metal.

How is acupuncture performed? This practice uses fine needles which are inserted into the skin of the patient particularly at the anatomical points of the body, in order to treat and prevent certain diseases. Proponents of this concept believe that the occurrence of diseases or ailments to individuals is due to some imbalance in their life force, otherwise referred to as Qi. The concept considers the existence of 14 channels that flow in the human body that branch out to the body's organs and systems. These channels are called meridians. If any of these channels are obstructed, ailments occur.

The practice of acupuncture incorporates the concept of Yin and Yang as well. Yin and Yang may cause varieties of imbalances in the Qi. If there is harmony between the two, the person's life force is considered normal. Once, there is imbalance between Yin and Yang, acupuncture is the remedy to achieve balance once again. The restoration is performed by stimulating the patient's acupuncture points in order to balance, adjust and harmonise the Qi.

Practitioners also use pressure, heat, friction and impulses of electromagnetic energy in order to perform stimulation of the anatomical points; through this technique the balance of the movement of energy in the body of the patient is achieved.

Sonopuncture and acupressure are some techniques in the practice that do not use needles. Sonopuncture uses ultrasound devices to create sound waves which will be applied to the anatomical points of the body. Others use vibration devices like tuning forks. On the other hand, acupressure uses finger techniques that relieve body pains. This remedy can be utilised with other manual techniques in healing or can also be used by itself.

Electromagnetic energy can produce impulses which can be applied to our bodies that produce tiny electrical discharges which can induce the maturity, growth and function of certain cells in our body. Practitioners need to insert needles in these areas; the impulses can further alter and stimulate the neurotransmitters in the body of the patient, making him or her feel better after having the treatment applied. This technique can be used for testing and diagnosis purposes.

The World Health Organisation (WHO) has identified the ailments to which acupuncture can be applied. The list includes common colds, acute bronchitis, toothache, cataracts, hiccups, gingivitis, constipation, ulcers, migraine, headache, diarrhoea, osteoporosis, Meniere's disease and many others. Chronic pain conditions and mind-body ailments are the most common illnesses treated by acupuncturists in the US.

However, patients must be wary about some risks that may occur when undergoing acupuncture treatments, such as hematoma, pneumothorax and HIV. If the needle is pierced into a circulatory structure, hematoma may result, if the needle is pressed too deep, a pneumothorax could be possible, while the patient may be at risk from HIV if the needles are not sterilized properly.

Remember, acupuncture is not an appropriate medical treatment; it is a sheer alternative remedy. One should still consult a physician who has the expertise to identify severe forms of ailments or illnesses.

Types of Acupuncture

For patients who opt for an acupuncture treatment, there are different types to choose from. These types may differ in one way or another; they still aim for the same objective; that is to provide relief from pain or certain diseases in patients.

Amongst the different types of acupuncture are TCM, various Japanese styles, French energetic, Korean hand, Auricular, Myofascially-based acupuncture, Impulses of electromagnetic energy, Sonopuncture and Acupressure.

TCM acupuncture uses the principles of complementary opposites in order to create balance in the body. TCM incorporates the principles of internal/external, yin/yang, hot/cold and excess/deficiency.

There are also different Japanese styles of acupuncture or otherwise known as "meridian therapy" that puts emphasises on feeling meridians during diagnosis and utilising the needling technique as well.

The French energetic technique is commonly used by MD acupuncturists; they put emphasis on meridian patterns specifically on the yin-yang pairs.

Another type of acupuncture is the Korean hand technique which is based on the principle that concentrations of Qi are found in the hands and feet of the person, making it effective for the entire body to receive acupuncture needles to those parts of the body.

When it comes to auricular acupuncture, needles are placed on particular points of the ear in order for certain addiction disorders to be treated. This technique believes that the microcosm of the body is the ear of the person.

Myofascially-based acupuncture is a technique which involves searching tender points in the meridian lines where the abnormal energy flows, that is where the needles are placed. This type of acupuncture is commonly utilised by physical therapists.

There are also acupuncture techniques which use impulses of electromagnetism, since the person's body produces tiny electrical discharges that induce the functions, maturity and growth of particular types of cells. Needles are inserted on areas where these certain types of cells are found. The impulses stimulate and change the neurotransmitters in the body which results in better feelings for the patient after the treatment. This technique is also used for diagnosis and testing purposes.

Meanwhile, some forms of acupuncture do not make use of needles, like sonopuncture and acupressure. Sonopuncture utilises an ultrasound device to create sound waves and transmit it to the parts of the body of the patient receiving treatment. Other practitioners of sonopuncture use other vibration devices such as tunings forks. On the other hand, in acupressure, hands are mainly used in providing relief to patients who are suffering from pain. Practitioners may use this technique on its own or opt for some other healing technique, which can be applied manually.

Nevertheless, the condition of the patient should be the basis of how many treatments he or she needs. The average number of treatments range from ten to fifteen which are undertaken for two to three times a week. Patients may spend $40 to $150; however, there are some insurance companies and HMO which offer whole or partial coverage. So, if you are interested, check if this procedure is included in your policy.

Acupuncture can be good for anyone who wants to relieve or prevent pain except for pregnant women. Practitioners decline to provide this technique if the woman is pregnant, but can continue again once she gives birth.

Taking herbs is also part of the treatment. If you have no idea about the quality of these herbs, ask your local doctor first before taking to ensure that they are safe, as contra-indications may occur if you are taking some medications at the same time.

When deciding which acupuncture is properly suited for you, remember it is your choice. Actually, all these types are effective, you just have to ask your doctor about the nature of the treatment as well as conduct some research to be aware of the causes and effects of the treatment being applied. Nevertheless, the application of the technique is painless, so allow the professional acupuncturist to do the rest, you just need to relax. Moreover, similar to conventional medicine, avoid expectations about overnight improvement; keeping an open mind takes time.

Acupuncture Closely Revealed

The significance of a person's chi in upholding bodily and mental health is the foundation of acupuncture. A person's chi is believed to exist in every living creature and it runs in the body following specific pathways. If the chi is blocked, then that is when health problems occur which result in persistent headaches, fever, weakness, muscles pain or worst and serious health conditions.

A Deeper Explanation of Acupuncture

The philosophy and practice of acupuncture began in ancient China. During the Old Stone Age of China, stones were designed into knives for medical purposes. This happened more than ten thousand years ago. Several years later, in the era of New Stone Age, needles were eventually made from stones aimed to be utilised for similar therapeutic purpose. It was found and proved further when stone needles of the same type were unearthed which were believed to exist during the New Stone Age.

Basically, the chi runs continuously throughout the 14 pathways of the body. The pathways are referred to as meridian points. There is a need of balance between the force of yin and yang so that the course of the chi will run through the body without any obstruction. Yin and yang is an ancient

Chinese philosophy that represents the strengths of the universe – yin embodies feminine strengths, while yang represents the masculine. It is believed that everything in the universe has both yin and yang to attain harmony.

Nevertheless, chi cannot liberally flow through the body if yin and yang are not balanced. Thus, the meridian points through which pathways of chi flow, have to be stimulated. Stimulation is done through inserting thin hair-like disposable needles in particular areas of the body to influence the harmony of the body and to provide healing.

For excellent therapy sessions, patients should consult a certified and trained acupuncturist who has the ability to carry out superior treatments. To be certified, the practitioner has to undergo training and obtain a license. Nevertheless, you have to be careful in choosing a t proficient practitioner who has enough practice to preclude the possibility of jeopardising the effect of the entire procedure. Today, it is important to verify the credentials of the practitioner to make sure an effective and safe treatment will be achieved.

What This Ancient Method Does

Relaxation is the foremost effect that a patient will encounter after the treatment. As frequently pinpointed, stress is considered as the main precursor of physical ailments. When the treatment is introduced to certain points of the body where relaxation and harmony flows, it may result in the patient becoming more at ease after stimulation.

Aside from relaxation, through acupuncture, pain control is increased. Although, in the course of the session, patients will normally feel minimal pain while the thin needles are inserted through the body in a gradual manner. The depths of placing needles vary on most cases which depend on the health requirements of the patient. The patient will feel pressure pain as the needles are inserted into the right depth; however, the whole procedure is not necessarily painful.

This technique is also recommended for patients who suffer from chemotherapy fatigue and nausea as well as pain after undergoing surgical operations. It was also found that this technique is greatly effective for migraines, back pains and menstrual cramps.

Variations of Conventional Acupuncture

Conventional acupuncture varies; these include auriculo-therapy and staple-puncture. Auriculo-therapy, otherwise known as ear acupuncture, is a practice which believes that the map for all main organs of the body is found in the ear. Therefore, in this technique, needles are placed in certain points around the ear and ear cartilage in order to treat particular organs like kidneys, liver or heart. On the other hand, staple-puncture is usually utilised in smoking cessation. The technique places staples on any parts of the ear area for a certain period in order to provide stimulation.

Undoubtedly, there is increasing evidence which proves that the alternative Oriental practice can compete with any modern form of treatment. This traditional practice may be good for the many people who are seeking an extensively recognised and long-established therapy. Acupuncture may be an alternative treatment for any one.

Things You Should Know About Acupuncture

In the practice of acupuncture, there are some things that people need to know ahead of time.

First, acupuncture provides holistic health care through the use of needles, which are inserted into certain points of the body. Research studies have been performed and the results prove that treatment can be provided to any part of the body which suffers disorders such as, ear, throat, nose, and eye as well as respiratory, gastrointestinal, nervous and muscular systems.

This technique makes use of very small needles and patients may possibly experience a slight twitch as the needle is inserted. The needles are carefully pressed from ¼ inch to 1 inch deep and will be placed there for 45 minutes to an hour depending on the health condition of the patient.

The patient will feel distension, cramping or electric tingling or even sensation if the needle is properly inserted. This implies that the treatment is producing positive effects.

It is required that needles used during acupuncture are clean and disposable especially in the US. This requirement aims to prevent patients from being contaminated by certain communicable diseases such as HIV or hepatitis.

Because this alternative treatment has been practiced for more than 2000 years, practitioners have developed a variety of acupuncture styles. Therefore, before you undergo a session, it is wise to be aware of the technique utilised and its consequences.

Look for an acupuncturist with proper training. Ask them where they obtained their training and their years of practice, as well as the situations they encountered when they carry out acupuncture as treatment for your condition.

Inquire about the credentials of the practitioners and what school provided them with their training and whether or not they possess a state board licence. If the state you live in does not require a licence, ensure that they can show some certificates confirming that they have the authority to practice their profession from the National Commission for the Certification of Acupuncturists.

The length of the treatment may vary in accordance to the characteristics of the ailment or disorder. Some problems are easy to fix, others may take time, such as alcohol and drug users who may stop their vices after 3 to 4 months. For those suffering from autism, treatment may last years since no cure for this illness is known as of yet.

Prior to treatment, you need to submit yourself first for physical examination and answer some questions before the insertion of needles is performed. There is nothing to worry about if the practitioner is good in their trade, however, safety precautions must be observed. This is a painless procedure. When needles come off, patients may find some spots of blood, any concerns about this have to be consulted with the specialist so that necessary medication can be prescribed.

Most commonly, after the first session patients will feel quick relief but others may not have the same experience. Thus, some treatments may last, on average, about 12 to 15 times. In a week, it is possible for a patient to undergo 2 to 3 sessions.

Follow-up sessions are advisable, especially if you find that the technique works for you. Follow-up sessions can be carried out twice in every 2 weeks or every month. The choice is yours. Keep in mind that you also need to consult your regular doctor who will help you to monitor the development of your condition.

The Effectiveness of Acupuncture

Painkillers are usual medications to people who want to attain relief whenever they are suffering from discomfort they are experiencing. Apparently, those painkillers reduce or remove the pain; however, they also bring about many side effects at the same time, resulting from the foreign chemicals introduced into your body. Today, modern medicine continues to develop drugs that can remove or reduce the pain in a much quicker manner, but do you think these quick pain relievers you are taking are really good for your health? Perhaps, it is wiser to try something more secure and effective like acupuncture.

Understanding Acupuncture

For the last few decades, acupuncture has risen in popularity. It was brought on through a recent trend in health. It is popularly known as a traditional Chinese practice on alternative medical treatment being observed as a homeopathic method of treatment. Apparently, acupuncture has gained a good reputation and is not considered as a quack treatment since scientifically inclined practitioners do not raise disapproval on alternative medicine. However, it is wiser for the patient to be aware of the technique to be applied to his or her condition and the consequences that may take place thereafter.

What is the Basic Procedure?

The procedure includes the insertion of needles into the skin of the patient. Each of these needles corresponds to a single point of the many pressure points positioned in the whole body. The Traditional Chinese Medicine proclaims that through the insertion of each needle into those pressure points, the practitioner can stimulate the life force or flow of chi which may result in relief of pain and eventually treat the ailment of the patient. Some would consider chi as a rubbish concept but, science suggests the idea that when needles are inserted into those points, endorphins or the natural painkillers of the body are released, which helps in relieving the pain. Acupuncture has various types of techniques; however, it is patient who will choose the technique after consulting the doctor and taking into account his or her health conditions.

Instruments Used

Today, modern practitioners of acupuncture are using fine and disposable stainless steel needles. The needles measure 0.007 to 0.020 inches in diameter and they must be sterilised using autoclave or ethylene oxide. Hypodermic syringe needles can be painful if poked into the skin of the patient but needles used for acupuncture relatively produce no pain for the reason that they are designed much finer compared to the hypodermic needle. To make the needle easier and sturdier to handle or hold, the upper third of the needle is enclosed in a thick wire made of bronze or plastic. The length of the needle and the depth of its insertion into the skin of the patient would likely depend on the specialist and his or her practice, to the style of the treatment. Other types of acupuncture do not make use of needles; rather, they use some devices to perform stimulation on certain areas where those needles are supposed to be placed. Nevertheless, these various types have the same aim, to relieve patients from pain and treat their ailments as well.

A Treatment Sample

Suppose a patient is suffering from a headache, she is diagnosed and treated. Stimulations are applied on her sensitive points, which are positioned at the webs between the palms and thumbs. Under the theory of acupuncture, these points are linked to the head and face of the individual, where treatment can be applied to relieve headaches and other ailments. As the needles are inserted into the skin of the patient, she will experience twinge, commonly accompanied by minor involuntary twitching of the area. While the treatment is applied, there are some things that may happen including:

- Awareness to pain. You may become sensitive to ache in the areas where the needles are placed or inserted.

- Indication of nausea. Nausea may arise if the treatment is employed to people with bad headaches.

- Quick relief. Some patients can experience some near-immediate relief from headaches.

Development

Acupuncture is an ancient method. It has intersected into the era of modern medicine with technology implementations and findings of recent scientific data. This technique usually used needles in treating, but as of today, electrical stimulations have become one of its common techniques of acupuncture practice, seeking to generate more effective results. As the treatment further enhanced, specialists of this field have combined eastern methods with western techniques. Some acupuncturists stick with the common methods of inserting needles, but others have tried to incorporate other useful and safe devices or manual techniques.

The practice started with one school of thought however, acupuncture practitioners realised that leaning on this one idea prevents progression. Thus, with the willingness to move towards a bright future, they look towards other horizons as well, thus acupuncture has been developed into different types of methods, which aim toward the same results, to relieve patients from pain and cure their illnesses.

Feedback and Studies

For some, the practice of acupuncture is not impressive. There are doubts or indifferences on oriental methods of treatment, which can be observed for the most part of the western medical profession. On the same note, others have driven the method down into the earth with brutal disparagement and disapproval. Better yet, in some recent studies and research, the efficacy (or insufficiency thereof) of the practice of acupuncture has been revealed. Meanwhile, some studies show that more research has to be conducted, although acupuncture has proven actual positive effect on some people, it was also found that treatment is not successful in all kinds of ailments which it claims to cure.

Apparently, despite the indifference and doubts of others, there are still doors open for the new age of acupuncture. Acupuncture is already a part of the alternative medicine, which is effective and safe to undertake for some people. You may give it a chance, when you achieve relief from body pains, you will not be displeased. For the reason that the Chinese have applied the technique for so many centuries, we may opt to this practice too.

Things to Consider When Undergoing Acupuncture

Some factors have to be considered by patients prior, during and after. Similar to this, acupuncture has a list of dos and don'ts for those who want to undergo this treatment and enjoy the benefits.

First, eating a large meal prior to the treatment or after is not allowed.

Avoid performing too much exercise or drinking alcoholic beverages 6 hours prior to treatment and after as well, avert yourself from engaging in sexual activity for the time being.

You have to fix your schedule prior to the session because it may take 45 minutes to 2 hours for one session to finish, therefore, give yourself time to rest before the schedule. However, the duration of treatment may depend on how many times you visit the clinic.

If you consulted a regular doctor before you went to your acupuncturist, do not forget to take the medications that were prescribed to you.

If after one or two sessions improvements are not yet experienced, write down the things you are experiencing. When you go went back to your acupuncturist, share the things you wrote down. You can then discuss modifications that should be done in the future to address those problems.

Taking herbal supplements may be incorporated by your acupuncturist while you are undergoing sessions, but if you do not know what side effects may occur when you take it together with your present medications, there could be a need to consult your doctor to know if consuming both will be safe for you.

Pregnant women are advised not to go through acupuncture procedure; however, they can always come back to their sessions once the baby is already delivered.

The developments of the treatment will take place depending on the performance of the specialist. Thus, it is wise to take into consideration their years of experiences and their skills in this field. This way you can feel assured they will find your correct diagnosis and proper acupoints where needles may be placed.

So, in looking for a skilled acupuncturist, we need to consult our regular doctors beforehand for their referral. It would also help to do a little research online. Apparently, there are roughly 3,000 acupuncturists in the country, so it should not be too difficult to find one.

Nevertheless, prior to making a decision to start the session with an acupuncturist, talk with your specialist about their credentials. Through this conversation, you will find out how much you will spend for the charge, this may range from $45 to more than $100 for every session. To have more knowledge about the expertise of the specialist, you can also ask about his or her previous clients. Ask for their names and contact numbers. If you find out that the service of the specialist will not work for you, do not hesitate to find another specialist who can offer and do a better job.

Remember that while you are going through a session, you need to relax. Tell the specialist if you experience itching or burning sensations or if you feel nervous, so that the specialist will remove the needles.

With these dos and don'ts in mind, ponder if it is proper for you to undergo this form of treatment. Thus, if ever conventional medication does not work, you could always make the decision to try acupuncture.

Eight Myths about Acupuncture

Acupuncture is surrounded by a lot of myths. Some of these myths are factual; others are ridiculous, while the remaining ones are considered half-truth. Reading the information below, will help you to understand which ones are reliable.

Myth #1: Acupuncture draws out pain. This is a myth. Those who claim that the procedure is painful are those who may have felt a tiny prick, compared to other who didn't feel any pain. Actually, when the needles are inserted through the skin or pulled out, no damage on the tissue is made. There are only a few uncommon cases where traces of bruises are found.

Myth #2: Patients can become infected by diseases like AIDS or hepatitis. This is only possible if the used needles are not sterilized. However, this does not happen in the US since practitioners are required to utilise needles which are disposable in order to avoid risk of those communicable diseases.

Myth #3: Acupuncture is a treatment for pain. This myth is only a half-truth. This holistic technique is proven not only for treating pain, it can also help the patient to stop addiction, prevent particular ailments and lose weight.

Myth #4: Most people believe that only Asians can practice acupuncture. This is a myth. Ever since 1952, 50 schools across the country provide trainings to students for this practice and eventually become licensed acupuncturists. This implies that any individuals who desire to learn this technique may have the chance to do so and assist patients in treating their diseases. To date, there are about 3,000 acupuncture practitioners working in the US.

Myth #5: Alternative medicine has no potential, according to medical doctors. This is untrue. These days more doctors have opened their minds to alternative medicine, believing that there are other options in treating patients apart from conventional medicine. The truth of the matter is, some doctors recommend acupuncturists to their patients if they find out that the treatment they have provided is not effective.

Myth #6: Patients will go through the four needle technique. This is another myth. The four needle technique will only be utilised by the specialist as a last resort if he or she feels that the patient's energy is not moving virtually.

Myth #7: Medical doctors should perform the procedure of acupuncture. This is erroneous. The training of doctors is very much different from that provided to acupuncture practitioners. Nevertheless, students have to be trained for 3,000 hours before they are issued a licence and allowed to practice their profession. So, for you to arrive at a better choice between a medical doctor and an acupuncturist, choose someone who has learned his or her practice for quite a long time.

Myth #8: Only third countries may opt for acupuncture treatment. This is another myth. Although the technique started in ancient China 2,000 years ago, the practice has been taught and learned in some of Asia's developed nations such as South Korea, Malaysia, Singapore and Japan.

In fact, acupuncture has been a practiced method for more than two decades in the United States. Thirty states allow the practice of this technique; twenty-two of them allow licensed professionals to practice after graduating from the training school and passing the required board examination of the state.

Although acupuncture has been performed by practitioners for a very long time now, there is still a necessity to opt for t this type of holistic healthcare which is the reason why this practice is taught in colleges and utilised today. The treatment is painless. A number of studies have revealed that the practice is efficient in curing various illnesses and preventing some of them from occurring.

Acupuncture is an Example of Holistic Healthcare

The ability to cure an illness by using alternative means refers to holistic healthcare. This method does not require any medication to be provided to the patient, however, treatment can be given using instruments, like needles.

Two thousand years ago, acupuncture began, only recently arriving to the US. According to studies, this practice is used for treating minor problems and preventing some others from occurring.

Needles utilised in the practice are very thin. They are smaller hypodermic syringe needles, very thing but thicker than human hair.

After one session, most patients who undergo the procedure will not experience significant changes, thus, patients need to continue attending a few more sessions. The good thing about this is the technique applied is not painful, so any sores will not be felt all over the body afterwards.

Several studies have been conducted about acupuncture in the UK, all producing positive results. There are 400 participants who claimed that they felt better after suffering from migraines when they underwent 3 months' worth of acupuncture treatment sessions. Meanwhile, in the US, because the needles help the body to fight against chronic pain and illness, the effect of acupuncture is more so proven in helping patients to deal with arthritis. The technique is not only effective, but is also cheaper than conventional medicine.

However, this holistic form of healthcare is more than just relieving people from pain of arthritis or migraines. According to clinical tests, it can also assist obese people in losing weight as well as those who need treatment because of insomnia.

In some countries, patients who do not have the ability to tolerate regular anaesthesia use acupuncture; the technique is a replacement to chemical anaesthesia applied before surgical operations.

It was also proven to help patients who battle against addictions, for instance drugs, alcohol and smoking. In a study conducted, smokers proclaimed that after just one treatment the average patient reduced half of the number of cigarettes they usually consume. Just imagine what they may be able to accomplish after even more sessions.

With this fact, more and more clinics have been established across the nation using acupuncture as another method of rehabilitation.

In the US, patient's pay their specialists anywhere from $75 to $150 for every session, yet acupuncturists charge lower than this as the treatment continues. Usually, a person will undergo 10 to 15 treatments, 2 to 3 times a week; however, the number of sessions actually depends on the patient's condition.

Check your insurance to see if this treatment is covered before undergoing the procedure. If you find that it is not included in the policy, perhaps it would be better to suggest its inclusion because it is way much cheaper than opting for a surgery.

Nevertheless, keep in mind the risks that come with the treatment if you decide to go through with acupuncture. To prevent this from happening, it is wise to choose a licensed specialist who can assure you that the needles are sterilized before they are applied to your body.

Actually, many professionals in the field of medicine recognise the effectiveness of alternative medicine. They often refer their patients to acupuncture practitioners when they find it could be beneficial for the patient.

Thus, if you are one of those people who are tired of suffering side effects from undergoing conventional medicine, it may be better to try a form of holistic healthcare and see what acupuncture can offer you. It may be a good choice among the many options you have, to help you deal with a chronic condition. The good thing about acupuncture, it is cost-effective and a painless treatment.

Understanding Acupuncture Energy

To understand this alternative form of healthcare, it is important to know the basic concepts of the practice in order to be educated about the whole process, which is referred to as "Qi." Qi occurs where the body possesses energy. At times, a person's Qi is troubled when the body confronts negative energies like illness or disease. Needles are positioned in certain points of the body to allow the flow of the Qi. Those points where the needles are placed will be stimulated thereafter. Some types of acupuncture make use of vibrating devices or a manual technique to perform stimulation. It is the task of the acupuncturist or therapist to determine the acupoints of the patient. After determining those points, needles will be inserted on top of the skin in order to unblock the factors or negativities that disrupt the Qi. For beginners, understanding the concept of Qi is not easy, thus, it would be wise to break each concept down to gain a better understanding.

The energy of the Qi is classified into five key types. These five key types are Jing, Qi, Xue, Shen Qi and Jin Ye.

In the English language, Jing would mean "essence," however, there is no corresponding terms for Jing in Western countries. Apparently, Jing can be inherited similar to DNA. Through Jing, individuals will have the ability to make their own energy through breathing air and eating specific foods. Jing is associated with "health" because a person hereditarily obtains certain health predispositions as well as makes lifestyle choices that will affect their health and the well-being of their children.

Qi is closely translated to "matter-energy" that causes the motion of the Universe; others associate Qi to the soul. Nevertheless, Qi is an important part of a person's good health.

Meanwhile, Xue is literally translated as blood, however, it is a type of energy that runs in the blood and passes through the energy of the body or Qi. Thus, the wellness of the two depends on one another. On the other hand, Shen Qi refers to the body's spirit. According to traditions, a person's spirit is found in the heart.

Finally, Jin Ye is another tangible concept that pertains to the fluids of the body, which include milk, saliva, genital secretions, tears, stomach fluids, sweat, and many other bodily fluids.

People would sometimes experience imbalance in their body due to imbalances in the flow of the Qi. Thus, if you are looking for ways and means to treat negative energies, acupuncture can help. Besides this alternative form of procedure also allows the patient to have a healthy body. Our body needs energy every day to perform our daily tasks. In addition, energies help us fight against illnesses, improve the heat of the body, develop and build on, manage the organs and blood of our body, break down and change the metabolism of our body. Therefore, opt for a procedure that is performed on a regular basis. Through this, you will be free from all of the negativities residing within your Qi.

The Soothing Effects of Acupuncture

Acupuncture has been around for more than a thousand years. This form of ancient Chinese medicine is commonly utilised for treating body pains. However, its coverage is not only for pain relief, rather its range has become wider and today it has been used to treat addictions, injuries, and also for disease prevention. Thus, if you entertain the idea of undergoing acupuncture for your health needs, below are some of the many benefits that many patients acquired from this treatment.

Pain

The technique is commonly used in helping patients to treat the body pains they suffer, particularly, arthritis and muscular pains. Apparently, there is a unique procedure for every type of arthritis. On that note, healing effects may also vary from one person to another. For those who have arthritis, if you opt for acupuncture, you have to go through several sessions, thus your cooperation with your specialist is a must requirement to achieve best results.

In addition, migraines, severe headaches, backaches, neck and shoulder aches, leg pains, muscle related injuries, trapped nerves, carpal syndrome, after surgery pains, sports injuries, toothaches, abdominal pains, menstrual pains and rheumatic pains are the other pain related illnesses which can be dealt with by acupuncture.

Depression

For symptoms of depression and anxiety, which include insomnia, suicidal tendencies, and loss of interest in social activities, acupuncture is highly recommended. It is believed that through this form of holistic healthcare, stress will be relieved and the flow of energy will improve, fighting against the causes of depression. Normally, improvements may manifest right after the first session. According to experts, acupuncture is a beneficial complement to other therapies used in treating depression like psychological counselling. Also, this technique improves wellness and health compared to chemical alternatives like antidepressants.

Insomnia

Instead of taking sleeping pills, acupuncture treatment has become a well-liked alternative remedy to insomnia. This technique works well at the nerve levels which relax and sooth your senses. Also, it is believed that this technique is a safer method of treating insomnia for the reason that it will bring you back to your natural cycle of sleeping, not by using chemicals, which may become an addiction. The good thing is, improvements may take place right after the first session. However, you still have to go through treatments within a stretched out period of time up to the moment that your natural sleeping cycle is restored.

Infertility

For people with fertility problems, acupuncture can be used as a complementary treatment to those who are going through other treatments, particularly women. Through this technique, women who suffer anxiety while undergoing treatments of fertility will achieve relief. This is proven successful in aiding patients who go through in-vitro fertilisation. To add, miscarriage rates have decreased for women who opt for acupuncture.

Others

Here are some more facts about ailments which acupuncture can treat:

- Bowel or bladder ailments which include pain or difficulties while urinating or if patients have urinary infections.

- Problems during menopausal periods, such as infertility, hot flashes and premenstrual tension.

- Disorders in the digestive system which include indigestion, nausea, diarrhoea and heartburn.

- Problems in the respiratory system such as hay fever, rhinitis, rashes and ulcers, eczema, prickly heat, and some types of psoriasis and dermatitis.

- Eye and mouth conditions such as dry eyes, cataracts, retinitis, conjunctivitis, post extraction pains and toothaches.

- Problems that arise during hot seasons such as stroke recovery, poor circulation and hypertension.

- Addictions, which include drinking, smoking and other heavy drugs.

If you suffer any of the above mentioned, surely, acupuncture is the best remedy for you. You need not worry because aside from the fact that it upholds health and wellness, it is harmless because it is a chemical-free alternative type of medicine compared to the traditional medical treatments.

What Do Acupuncturists Do?

An acupuncturist is someone who practices acupuncture. Most of the specialists in the area of alternative medicine utilise needles or some instruments, which usually depend on the type of acupuncture treatment that will be applied to help the body achieve balance and harmony.

However, before the specialist can go on with the procedure, patients will be asked a few questions. Then, patients will often undertake a physical examination that includes pulse checking, and observing the shape, coating and colour of tongues. In addition, the texture and colour of your skin will be checked as well as your posture to find out clues about your state of health.

After the preliminary check-ups, you will be instructed to lie down on the examining table, which is usually padded, and then some needles will be inserted into your skin. Compared to other needles, the type of needle used is different because it jiggles and twirls as it is pushed further into the skin.

Sometimes, you will not feel the needles at all. At times when you do, you will only feel a slight twitch that will disappear in a little while. When all of the needles are placed in their proper positions, they remain there for 15 to 60 minutes. Most of the time, you feel relaxed which allows will allow you to doze off into a sound sleep. After the completion of the treatment session, the removal of needles will follow and you will be allowed to leave or go home.

There are cases where acupuncture is found to be more effective if the needles are heated first. This method is called moxibustion, when the therapist gets a small bunch of dried herbs and lights it. The dried herbs or moxa, also called mugwort, is held above the needles as it gradually burns and produces a small smoke with a pleasant and incensed smell; however, the lighted herb will not directly touch your body.

Another method is electrical acupuncture. This makes use of electrical wires, which are hooked to the needles. A weak current will flow through it, but it will not cause any sensation, not even a little.

There are also times that the acupuncturist specialist will prescribe herbal medications as you go through the treatment session;

this will also aid in making the treatment effective and successful.

Ensure that the person conducting the treatment is a licensed acupuncturist. Acupuncturists complete a four year training at an accredited college of oriental medicine before they can obtain a licence. In some states like California, the California Acupuncture Committee is the governing body that awards the title to qualified specialists in this area of study.

Another organisation that awards the same title is the national Certification Commission for Acupuncture and Oriental Medicine. Practitioners who obtained their licence from this organisation are required to display its copy inside their clinics or offices.

Aside from taking into consideration the credentials of the acupuncturist, there are some important things you need to ask which include the styles used in completing the procedure since there are techniques which do not utilise needles in treating a patient. While no studies have proven that one technique is more effective than the other, there are some patients who are at ease with one style instead of the other.

You should also inquire and discuss further about the duration of the treatment. In some cases, there are patients who suffer from chronic pain or illness that need to wait a period of months in order to see if he or she has achieved some improvements. Knowing these facts will help you plan and organise your schedule since you will be visiting the clinic anywhere from two to three times a week.

Similar to a medical doctor, acupuncturists are just around to help you get well; however, if you do not find any progression with his or her style of treatment, it might be time to get another opinion.

Is Acupuncture the Remedy For You?

As the acceptance of alternative medicine grows in Western culture, acupuncture has become one of the popular practices. Since it quickly rose in popularity, more and more patients are choosing this practice instead of opting for to western medicine to cure body pains and stress and to uphold a person's overall wellbeing. If you are pondering about attempting to undergo acupuncture but still questioning if it is safe or proper option for you, here is some information which may help you in making a more informed decision.

Description and Origin

The practice of inserting thin hair-like needles into particular points of the body for healing purposes, pertains to acupuncture. In theory, these particular points are referred to as "acupuncture points" which are located along the pathways of the body where vital energy is supposed to run. Needles are used to allow unobstructed flow of energy because there is a possibility it may become stagnated. Today, the practice is known and applied in numerous Asian cultures; this includes Tibet, Japan, and Korea.

Nevertheless, China is the leading proponent of this practice.

Acupuncture in the Western World

The utilisation of acupuncture as a western method of medical practice is one of the largely debated issues between the Eastern and Western World. Although this form of alternative medicine has been practised as an effective technique in China for almost five thousand years, no concrete scientific evidence from studies or research can prove the healing composition of acupuncture.

According to sceptics, the good effects of this practice are plainly considered as placebo effects. On the other hand, believers of acupuncture claim that the effectiveness has not yet been proven; however, further research affirms that it is harmless and can be used as supplement to western medicine.

However, the FDA has not fully approved the standards of acupuncture because there are some unregulated techniques which continue to subsist, like re-using needles. Apparently, acupuncture certifications are used to make money on desperate patients whose western medical treatments have failed, making those certificates a sham. The practice as a means of treatment was even declared unproven by the National Council against Health Fraud because according to the council, it originated from primitive and false healing concepts.

Should You Try It

If there is one thing that Western science can agree with acupuncture, it is the fact that no study has proven that it has provided harmful effects. Because there are benefits evident, numerous physicians accept the fact that there is no reason why acupuncture should not be used if the medication provided is not injurious to the health of the patient. Also, scientists also would assert that it is because of the failure to conduct research that the therapeutic composition of acupuncture is not yet verified or established.

Today, the interest in the many forms of Chinese medication keeps growing despite the fact that it has been a debated issue in the Western world. Somehow, through the increasing recognition of the practice, its healing properties will be explored and discovered.

More Information on Acupuncture

If there are acupuncture centres in your community, helpful information about the practice may be obtained from these places. It would be easy for you to locate the nearest centres or find the most skilled acupuncturist when you search the Internet. Since centres are usually packed with long waiting lists, it would be wise to set an appointment to completely address necessary inquiries.

Thus, if you cannot obtain improvements through western medicine, try to look into another option. Perhaps acupuncture would be a great help as numerous people have discovered the benefits provided by this ancient alternative practice. It is harmless and safe, thus, there is nothing to lose, better yet, you can even improve your health.

Can Anyone Go For Acupuncture?

Similar to other medical practices, acupuncture can be practiced in a number of different ways. However, as an acupuncturist you have to be proficient in the field in order to practice. Equip yourself with helpful knowledge and skills on various techniques as well as specialised one-on-one techniques special to acupuncture. Keep in mind that this procedure may not be effective for everyone, at the same time not all techniques are appropriate for each patient. It is important that as a professional acupuncturist, you find the best technique for each patient and the condition they are suffering from. Most of the time, acupuncture is good for treating headaches, stomachaches, infertility, arthritis, back pains and other conditions and diseases. In some cases, this practice can help patients in times they are in pain, as well as correcting some imbalances in the flow of the Qi, or energy flow.

When you hear of acupuncture, most of the time you associate it with the traditional Chinese practice. During treatment you may be advised to lie on your stomach or sit in a comfy chair. While doing so, the acupuncturist will place needles which are as a thin as hair, into your body. Needles are inserted on certain spots, referred to as meridians. The needles will stimulate the body to induce energy flow throughout. In the practice of acupuncture, energy flow is often referred to as Qi. This practice has been popularly utilised all over the world as well as in the United States. With the use of acupuncture you can help release negative energies from your body in an alternative way.

There is also the slightly different technique introduced by Japanese acupuncturists. If you choose Japanese acupuncture, you may say it is less rigorous and intrusive compared to the other techniques. Most patients find the Japanese technique more appealing and pleasing since it makes use of shorter and thinner needles. Only few needles are used generally.

Another acupuncture technique is the Korean practice, which is ideal for people who have troubles with lying down and sitting for long periods of time. If you are a bit scared of the other methods of acupuncture, this technique is another good way to start. This technique targets the hand and fingers; treating more than arthritis as hands can affect the whole body. Learning these acupoints is similar to art, which is why Korean hand therapists are considered to be the most skilled acupuncturists.

Aside from Japanese and Korean techniques, there is also auricircular acupuncture, which is performed in a single location of the body if needles cannot be placed into all points of the body. In auricircular acupuncture, needles are inserted close to the ears of the patients. Most of the time, this technique is ideal for alcohol and drug rehabilitation programmes.

Thus, for people whose conditions bring them pain, acupuncture could be a good alternative to help in that pain relief and treatment needed. To be sure that you choose the correct technique, talk to your acupuncturist about the procedure.

A Primer on Medical Acupuncture

Have you ever had a desire to be punctured by numerous needles? Your answer is probably no! Actually, this is the picture visualised by most people when they hear the word "acupuncture." Most people view this alternative practice with suspicion and downright terror, which is not surprising. Nevertheless, this rather painless procedure derived from the ancient Chinese, has helped patients to achieve relief from chronic pain symptoms. If used appropriately, it can be a great aid in controlling various medical conditions such as severe fatigue and pain.

How Does Needle Puncture Work?

Practitioners of acupuncture believe in the existence of energy flows. Energy, otherwise known in Chinese as Qi, travels all over the body of the person through pathways, which are called meridians. These pathways flow very near to the skin's surface in specific areas and can be reached by acupuncture needles. Similar to plumbing, if pipes are blocked or flow in the wrong pathway, health problems may arise. Thus, when needles are inserted into the skin of the patient, blocks will be released and the flow will become normal.

This principle of acupuncture may sound like a justification without basis, but actually there are many scientific studies that rationalize the effects of acupuncture. Despite the fact that there is no known and exact scientific basis, it was found that new theories give the impression that involvement of impulse modulation from nerve to spinal cord, complex neurochemical effects of the brain and changes in the microscopic connective tissue occur during acupuncture.

What Are The Concerning Risks and Side Effects?

It is not surprising to see that different medical practices are not always understood. For instance, the decades of using aspirin and penicillin is merely based on their beneficial effects, but doctors do not know their exact function. Nevertheless, safe use of the technique must be ensured too, in the same level as positive results.

Apparently, acupuncture may manifest some side effects too, like other methods utilised for the treatment of some medical conditions, such as infections and complication after surgeries as well as allergic reactions and side effects after taking medications. In the case of needle puncture, some risks include are injuries, minor bleeding, rare infections, dizziness and small bruises.

To minimise the probable risks and side effects; you have to look for a licensed specialist. In every country, there is a government office that regulates the issuance of licences or an organisation that implements the rules and regulations of the practice.

How Do Treatments Go?

The treatment sessions mostly start with the initial evaluation conducted by the acupuncturist on the medical and current bodily state of the patient. Palpitations on multiple pressure points are conducted and formulations of treatment regimen will be produced. Most treatment sessions are conducted from 10 to 20 times which may last from 30 to 90 minutes in a day. The acupuncturist will place the needles at the specific points in a careful manner and leave them for quite some time. Mild sensations are the most reported feeling while the puncture is being conducted; nevertheless, no real pain has ever experienced.

After you undergo the procedure, most commonly, you feel the exhaustion and are often in need of a rest. Others will experience a great improvement in the level of their energy. This means that responses vary depending on the individual who undergoes this method of treatment. For some people, a quick relief from symptoms is achieved. In some other cases, patients may notice improvements only after going through a few more sessions. But, you do not have to worry, just keep updating your acupuncturist about your state of health to make sure that things are working as anticipated.

The thought of needles should not frighten you because of the effective relief of pain that has been proved through the use of acupuncture. However, always bear in mind, it is a supplement to existing medical therapy and patients should not forget to continue their current medications or treatments.

Moreover, people around the world who suffer from severe diseases or ailments can now achieve the safe and effective application of this method, which used to be an exclusive Chinese therapy.

Acupuncture for All Those Simple Aches and Pains

At first, the thought of undergoing acupuncture treatment could seem scary, especially if you have a phobia of needles and injections, like me. You might think that this practice of sticking needles into your skin may not work for you. However, nevertheless, you cannot deny the fact that you have been suffering for quite a long time now from headaches or severe pains. Regular consultations to your doctor may not be providing you with the relief that you need. Perhaps, trying to visit an acupuncture therapist would be of great assistance. After all, who has not heard someone who is being tormented from pains of arthritis and continues to follow the medications prescribed by the doctor, but are not getting the relief that they need.

Now, you may be thinking if this kind of treatment would be effective for you. Since this treatment follows the traditional Chinese medicine principles and does not concur with the standards of modern Western medicine, you might feel a bit doubtful. Apparently, the procedure of using needles to treat people was discovered and used thousands of years ago in China, long before the inventions of x-rays or microscopes or prior to the discovery of germs and bacteria.

The fact that acupuncture has been utilised for thousands of years and is still being practiced today, proves its effectiveness. If you are considering acupuncture, this knowledge can assure your decision.

What Typically Happens When You Go To An Acupuncturist?

When you visit an acupuncturist, some inquiries should be conducted, including your medical history, your current state of health, and the symptoms of the ailment that you have; the characteristics of your tongue and face will also be observed by the specialist. It appears to some specialists that the person's tongue is the best indicator of state of health of your internal organs. They should also examine the sounds of your body, such as the sounds that come from your lungs. The smell of your body can be another indicator of your overall wellness which will be taken into consideration when the acupuncturist makes his diagnosis.

The treatment that is necessary for your body will depend on what the specialist discovers about your body. Since acupuncture is based on traditional Chinese medicine, the illness that occurs in your body is believed to be caused by some imbalances and loss of harmony among the organs of your body. Thus, there is a need to use needles, which will be inserted into the specific points of the patient to achieve once again, the balance that is needed by the body and organs.

The procedure will start by inserting very thin, hair-like needles into the proper positions of your body. As the insertion is performed, no pain can be manifested to the many people who undergo this treatment. In fact, the needles used by the specialist are usually very thin compared to the needles used for syringes. Most people claim that as the needles were inserted into their bodies, it helps them to attain calmness and relaxation.

How Does The Use Of These Needles Help You?

Through this practice, many ailments or illnesses have been effectively treated. These include common colds, headaches, arthritis, asthma, back pains and even infertility.

Acupuncture has been studied extensively by the experts of Western medicine despite the fact that it does not form part of Western medicine. According to some theories, the practice involves stimulation of the brain to release the natural painkillers of the body. Actually, the practice could also motivate the human body to attain proper circulation.

As of today, Western medicine continues to study the practice of this form of holistic health care, to determine the manner of incorporating it with practices of Western medicine. This is one reason why it is effective for some to undergo acupuncture as well as following any other medical practice their doctor may suggest.

In fact, it is harmless because it should not cause any hurt and may even aid you in achieving relief and wellness from the aches and pains that you have been suffering lately.

Acupuncture Could Help You Finally Manage Your Stress Levels

Today, busy people are experiencing a lot of stress. If you work too much without thinking of some ways to remove stress, it may cause danger to your body; you may get stress-related diseases. For some people, stress could be one reason why they suffer headaches or insomnia or worse yet, serious heart ailments.

Anti-stress pills may help your body to relax but it may cause some side effects. That is another worry for you as well as for me. Nevertheless, I have good news for you; why not try acupuncture. Undergoing this form of alternative medicine may actually relieve the stress you are suffering from. It is harmless to opt for this treatment, so if you want to be relieved from the ailments caused by stress, this could be one great way.

If you try acupuncture and find that it is not the right type of treatment for you, you can also stop.. But if you find it effective, you will be very happy to see the stress you are feeling starting to disappear. You will not be relying on pills or dangerous chemicals anymore.

How Will You Attain Relief With Those Needles Inserted Into Your Skin?

As we know, acupuncture originated from ancient Chinese traditional medicine, thus, its principles have depended on the theory that our bodies as well as our internal organs should maintain balance in order to keep ourselves in good condition. Thus, without balance due to our environment and lifestyle, illnesses will occur. Imbalances will also result in to stress, which is one reason why we can often find ourselves sick; we could be feeling irritable and tense. Oftentimes, we feel irritable and uneasy to relax.

When you undergo the procedure, needles will be inserted into some points of your skin. These needles will serve as a stimulation device that will rouse the nerves in your body. Once the nerves are stimulated, scientist claim it will transmit a message to the brain commanding it to release natural pain killers existing in your system. By the time the natural painkillers are released, you will feel relaxed and relieved from pain.

The needles also help the patients to achieve good circulation in the body. If you have good circulation, many toxins or waste will be removed from your body, cleansing your system and allowing you to attain a healthy body and organs. Oxygen will freely circulate from your lungs to your cells without any blockages. The result is a much healthier well-being or a better feeling for a longer period of time.

Acupuncture treatment sessions are similar to having massage therapy in a spa. A good massage helps you to have a relaxing sleep at night; it is the same with acupuncture. During the procedure of inserting the needles on the surface of your skin, as the right nerves are properly stimulated, you will also experience a soothing feeling resulting in a good relaxing sleep.

You may wonder how you can be relieved if you are pierced with numerous needles. Actually, you will not feel anything at all because these needles are too thin. Most of the time, patients' claim they feel a tingling as soon as the needles are inserted to their skin. Apparently, this is the sign that treatment is starting to work.

Through attending acupuncture sessions, you will have the ability to manage stress in a proper manner allowing you to live in a healthier lifestyle far from things that may cause chronic ailments, which usually occur due to stressful work in the office or serious personal or family problems. But remember, because you have one way of relieving your body pains does not mean you have to forget about consulting your regular doctor. Continue your regular tips to your physician as well as your medications. Consider acupuncture as one great complement to achieve a healthier well-being.

Facial Acupuncture

Everybody wants to look beautiful inside and out. We utilise a number of beauty regimens to maintain good looking skin and younger features. However, due to some hormonal issues, emotional changes or stress can make our features look worn out and exposes some lines or wrinkles. So, you really need to take care of yourself regularly. The good thing is, through facial acupuncture you can achieve and maintain a blooming appearance every day.

Facial acupuncture is a procedure, which uses painless mini needles applied on some points of your face to renew its features at the same time as improving your overall health. This technique is good for erasing bags under your eyes, as well as wrinkles, helping you to attain that younger look. It also helps clearing your face from acne and pimples.

Apparently, to achieve that impressive appearance, during the procedure, the fine needles will be placed on specific acupuncture points on the face, eyes, and neck in order to rouse the natural energies of the person. Most of the time, after the procedure you will achieve a better facial colour.

Anyone can undergo facial acupuncture because it is harmless and painless; preventing the signs of aging. However, for individuals who are pregnant or suffering from flu or colds, acute herpes or allergies, you have to wait until these circumstances are over.

Nevertheless, if you are not currently suffering from any of the above afflictions, you can opt to undergo the procedure anytime. First, you have to pass the evaluation process to be performed by the acupuncturist who will assess your age, diet and lifestyle. If you are in good shape, then sessions may proceed. You will probably go through a number of treatments, which may range from 12 to 15 times. Duration of the session may be prolonged if your skin manifest jowls, tends to sag or if you have weary eyes.

Treatment sessions may be performed two times every week, which may last from 45 minutes to an hour. If your schedule will not allow you to be present for two sessions every week; you can choose to be treated once in a week which may take 90 minutes. After attending your regular sessions, you have to come back to the clinic and undergo a follow up treatment, which will be conducted every 2 weeks in the following 2 months and once a month thereafter.

If some clinics use needles, others utilise herbs by forming them into poultices, masks or moisturizers. However, before using any of these, ask your regular doctor to ensure no allergic reactions will occur if you complement this technique with your regular medications.

Most of the time, improvements may be observed after the first facial acupuncture treatment. There will be an increased glow on your complexion which is usually referred to by the Chinese as improvement of the Qi or blood flow of your face. As the days wear on, it becomes more apparent. Wrinkles will disappear and skin will be more toned.

By the time you reach your fifth or seventh treatment session, you will see more evident improvements. You face will look more lightened, as if you just had a great vacation. Therefore, as soon as you finish the sessions, you will appear and feel younger by 5 to 15 years. Nevertheless, the impressive result may typically depend on the manner in which you take care of yourself after each session.

Overall, facial acupuncture is really a good procedure. It aids in the elimination of facial lines, reduction of wrinkles, and improvement of your facial colour because your skin will glow. Also, the tension of your face and furrows will be relaxed, eyes will brighten, dark circles are reduced and become less puffy, sagging skin will be toned, and natural radiance of the skin and eyes will be enhanced. The treatment will further result in slowing the aging process, promoting well-being and health, as well as revitalising your whole body.

So, what are you waiting for? Get that remarkable facial radiance and well-being through facial acupuncture. Look for a clinic now that offers great deals and service to their customers.

Acupuncture and Weight Loss

The number of overweight individuals continues to increase at an alarming rate. Many people reach levels of obesity that has to be treated through surgery. However, there might be an alternative method available in the form of acupuncture.

Acupuncture is a holistic form of healthcare that utilises needles in order to treat some ailments or disorders suffered by patients. If you are thinking of a balloon being popped by a needle blasting the air out, that will not happen to you. This procedure is harmless. Though the needles are applied or inserted on certain points, it is aimed to stimulate the nerves of the body allowing the release of endorphins, which will take over control of the appetite of the person.

However, prior to the application of the needles, the acupuncturist will have to evaluate the patient by asking a few questions and performing some examinations. Through the evaluation process, the acupuncturist will determine what the primary cause of being overweight is. Also, the examination of the patient will aid the acupuncturist in figuring out the points where the needles will be placed. It is essential that your pulse be determined to give the acupuncturist the general information about your energy rate and the wellness of your stomach.

The acupuncturist will also check your mouth, examining your tongue to see if you have any peeling or cracks. The puffiness of your stomach will also be checked as these factors will give clues or reasons why you are overweight.

When the specialist is sure of the reason, the needles will be placed on certain areas or parts of the body. He or she may use the multi-targeted approach which aims to lower the weight of the body through escalating the output of the pituitary gland. The specialist will insert the needles on the ear and in two areas of the three acupuncture points, including the stomach, mouth, lung, spleen, thyroid, endocrine or kidney.

The "Four Gate" points could be utilised to achieve circulation of energy through the entire body. This will be used during the initial treatment. To increase the release of endorphins and rouse metabolism, electro stimulation will be performed.

After placing the needles on the acupuncture points, the specialist will leave them inserted for thirty to forty-five minutes. Afterwards the needles will be removed and ear tacks with adhesive will replace the spot where the needles were inserted into your skin.

These ear tacks will do the job further by rousing the mild endorphins and releasing them, allowing the patient to relax and focus on their weight loss efforts. To release the needed endorphins, a mild pressure will be applied whenever the patient feels the hunger.

The patient has to do his or her part by reducing cravings of certain food or cutting down food intake. According to recent studies revealed, this procedure helps patients to lower their insulin levels or lipid levels.

The best thing about this procedure is there is no chance for any addiction to occur in the future, aside from the fact that it is proven to be harmless since it creates no side effects. What the patient needs to do is to continue his or her regular sessions towards the end and to keep a healthy diet and exercise because the function of the needles is only to control the weight.

However, patients must be reminded that the number of treatments may take quite some time since it will depend on the weight they would like to lose. The pace of their sessions will differ depending on how quickly or gradually they would like to lose the weight, as well as their level of commitment.

On average, if you would like to lose five to ten pounds, you must attend your sessions every two or three days. The number of treatments will be reduced later on, depending on the progress. Once results are seen, you can always opt to stop the treatment as well.

Nutrition and Acupuncture

Recently, there has been an increase in the number of people who want to undergo acupuncture treatment. One of the improvements that you will see through acupuncture is the ability to maintain a better diet. You start to believe that eating healthy food will help you to achieve effective results through acupuncture. All those unhealthy problems will start to clear up. Right before you finish your appointments with your acupuncturist, you can assure yourself that the treatment can help you have an entirely refreshed and healthier life. Once you start with a healthy diet, you will begin to feel a lot happier and healthier.

When you start an all-new programme for your diet, it would be better to consult a medical doctor beforehand, to learn any important information. If your doctor says it is healthy, you should feel assured and continue with your plans. You will also need to consult your acupuncturist about your new diet, and ask for their guidelines. Another thing to consider is consulting a professional prior to making any major diet changes; you want to make sure that you are making the right improvements. If you start to experience any tiredness, illness or weakness, always consult your doctor.
Herbal supplements are often recommended by acupuncturists to take along with

acupuncture treatment. They may provide you a tea to drink or herbal pill to swallow prior to the treatment session. It is very important to inform your acupuncturist if you have any allergies, or if you are taking any other medication. Therapists also sell tea bags, which you can also use at home, or they can recommend some foods that will also allow you to achieve the same effects. There is much evidence to support herbal medication in combination with acupuncture.

After maintaining a healthy diet, continuing acupuncture treatment, and taken herbal supplements you will start to notice a difference in the way you digest your food. These techniques will allow your body to utilise the good you consume at a good level. For instance, instead of eating food in large bites or a quick manner, you focus on chewing slowly before swallowing. Besides you opt to pay close attention to your food intake. Another healthy way of digesting your food is to avoid watching TV while eating. It is important to learn how to enjoy each bite you take. Following these techniques will help you concentrate the energy of your body to the stomach.

Watch your diet and the way you eat. Give emphasis to the things you need to consider as advised by your acupuncturist. If your therapist does not provide a more specific suggestion, try to ask for advice from your regular doctor about a healthy diet. It is important that you will attain great benefits both from a healthy lifestyle and acupuncture treatments.

Acupuncture Is Effective For Losing Weight

Our generation has regarded physical fitness as number one on the wellness list. People who choose to live a healthy lifestyle generally look for the most effective and newest method of losing weight. One way to do away with excess fat is acupuncture. The procedure involves inserting fine, filiform needles on specific acupuncture points of the body. According to studies, this procedure is a very effective way to lose weight.

You may think it sounds uncomfortable to have needles piercing your body as a means to reduce excess weight; but this method has been proven to control temptations of hunger over long periods of time

The Skinny on Acupuncture Weight Loss

In recent studies, it was determined that emotions usually affect the weight that people gain. When people are in need of comfort they may opt for a chocolate bar, fast food, even if they are not hungry. Oftentimes, gaining weight in an excessive level, is not a physical issue, it is actually an emotional issue. Without you knowing, you eat too much whenever you are pressured, upset, or stressed.

With acupuncture you can control the temptation to eat more food than your body needs. When the spots are stimulated, patients will attain remarkable balance of emotions and physical well-being. While the needles are inserted in those areas, some hormones will be released within the entire body, which will help you control hunger and manage the impulse of overeating.

How Acupuncture Brings About Weight Loss

When you undergo acupuncture for the purpose of losing weight, practitioners will aim acupuncture points behind your ear. As the needles are placed, the ear area will be stimulated resulting in the release of endorphins within your body, in a large quantity. These endorphins are referred to as feel-good hormones, which function as a natural fever and pain relievers. Like a good workout, having this acupuncture leaves you feeling renewed as endorphins are released.

Endorphins are body compounds that provide better relaxation to patients with considerable stress. Thus, when patients achieved wellness in their emotions, there is a great probability that losing weight will be successful while undergoing acupuncture. In fact, endorphins are regarded as a natural pain reliever.

Most of the acupuncture points are found close to muscle tissues and nerve endings. However, according to most patients of this alternative practice, they experience nominal pain or none at all. While the needles are inserted into the body, the nerves send signals to the brain to allow the pituitary gland to distribute those endorphins.

For better management of weight, acupuncturists may utilise the multi-targeted approach, but it depends on the requirements of the patients. This approach may stimulate those gateway points of the body in order to motivate a decrease in appetite of the patient, or decrease the body's retention of water.

Conferring with an Acupuncturist Specialist

Today, there are a number of acupuncture specialists who offer a number of different services. Ensure that you choose a specialist that is well trained and professional when you consider going through this type of treatment in the future, for purposes of losing excessive weight. Avoid poorly trained specialists who may not have the sufficient ability or skills to pinpoint the essential meridian points. If you settle for the least trained, chances are you will feel body pains and discomforts.

Furthermore, herbal supplements are often required by specialists to be taken to support good effects within a long-term period. These supplements will help you attain more benefits, which may result in the reduction of the extensive sessions you need to attend. Nevertheless, you still need to pay some visits to your specialist within the whole course of the treatment to monitor your status.

It may not be good to opt for strenuous workouts or crash dieting for the intention of losing weight. You can choose the successful and natural weight loss method through acupuncture, especially if a well-trained specialist conducts it. Though it may not be proven as a cure-all method, it can be the proper solution for you in order to lose that excess fat from your body and achieve a healthy lifestyle.

Acupuncture Can Help You Quit Smoking

Old habits die hard. If you have been smoking for a long time it can become very difficult to quit. However, there are many solutions that can help you break the habit, like gums and nicotine patches. If you would like to try an alternative and holistic solution to quit smoking, acupuncture can be very helpful.

Once you decide to seek acupuncture treatment to quit smoking, you need to be sure that you want to make the commitment. The specialist will ask some questions and carry out some examinations, including looking at your ears and finding spots where you have low energy.

After examining some areas of your body, the acupuncturist will identify the essential spots or acupoints where sharp, yet thin needles will be placed. In various acupoints, five needles will be inserted.

After the insertion of the needles, you will have to wait for about an hour for the procedure to be complete. When you are through, the specialist will remove the needles, and advise you to wear ear magnets, which will further continue the treatment. According to some smokers, while they go through the procedure they get sleepy or feel a prick on the surface of their skin, a very minimal and tolerable pain.

Patients who want to stop smoking needs to go to the clinic four to six times in order to obtain significant improvements. Actually, one research study revealed that after going through one or two sessions, patients claimed that they experienced a decline in the quantity of cravings to smoke. Eventually, after five to six sessions, seven out of ten patients were able to stop smoking entirely.

However, some people still doubt the effectiveness of this method, since research that has been conducted only used a small number of test subjects. Many of the studies show that although the treatment of smoking through acupuncture can show some immediate results, it may not work the same over longer periods of time.

On that note, you have to keep in mind that this method is temporary; it will only pave a way to start something which you have to conclude on your own. Most smokers who go to the clinic two or three times every week have to return again for some follow up sessions in the days or weeks to come.

Nevertheless, you have to look for ways to avoid the temptation of picking up a cigarette as you undergo the treatment. Do this by preventing yourself from going along with people who smoke, because you may surely be persuaded to smoke with them. You have to develop a personal mantra which will serve as your routine once the urge occurs.

Cravings may last for a short period of time, but it is important to discipline yourself and work hard towards a smoke-free lifestyle.

Licensed specialists for this practice are the only authorized people who should perform acupuncture treatment. To find out if the acupuncturist you have chosen is accredited by the National Commission for Acupuncture and Oriental Medicine, you can research about it online. Or you can ask your acupuncturist personally, if you'd like to find out about how much experience they have.

Settle for the best and a skilled specialist and if you found one, you have to prepare yourself too. You must establish your commitment to the programme since it is not only your acupuncturist who work on this, the treatment sessions also requires your cooperation in order for you to successfully give up the habit

Acupuncture has aided alcoholics and addicts cease their addictions, in the same manner, it can also help smokers. You may doubt it, but it might not hurt a try.

Bye-Bye Smoking! Hello Acupuncture!

One of the most renowned practices of treating the addiction of smoking is acupuncture. This alternative form of healthcare goes back as far as 3000 BC in the earliest era of China. This alternative treatment has been utilised for many therapeutic and medicinal purposes. Furthermore, studies have shown that this treatment has been an effective means of treating chronic smoking addiction and drug dependence.

Today, there are various quit-smoking cessation therapies and medication available, but acupuncture is the most recommended alternative method particularly if conventional medication does not work out successfully. To cure the condition in a more intense and emotional degree, the strategic placement of needles in certain areas of the body is used. Because, smokers have to liberate themselves from the psychological and physiological smoking addition, they need a more holistic form of treatment.

The strategic insertion of needles is usually performed behind the ear of the patient or on the ear cartilage area. This area is pinpointed as location where the calming effects occur to curb the cravings of smoking in the patient. When people are stressed, depressed or bored, most of the times they develop a smoking habit. Aside from the ear area, needles are also sometimes inserted in the wrists and hand of the patient to prop up a stable energy flow within the body. Once patients feel relaxed, they are able to focus their efforts on quitting.

Acupuncture can also help you in dealing with symptoms of withdrawal. To do away with discomfort and pain as you undergo the smoking cessation period, this alternative form of treatment will help you achieve increased tolerance in dealing with withdrawal symptoms such as mild to severe palpitations, nausea and dizziness. Often these withdrawal symptoms are what make people pick up the habit once again.

Cigarettes contain nicotine, a toxic and addictive substance. To most smokers, nicotine addiction is the biggest challenge, making quitting very difficult. If smokers do not have a steady stream on this addictive substance, they will often feel uncomfortable and depressed.

According to patients who went through acupuncture, cigarettes become unsatisfying as cravings are reduced. There are times that they promptly stop picking up a cigarette because it would leave a terrible taste in their mouths. To get rid of this terrible taste, they often eat lozenges or mints.

In a recent study of skilled practitioners, seven out of ten smokers were able to successful quit smoking after two to three weeks. Meanwhile, other patients were unable to fight back the habit totally, better yet it is still significant to note that their cigarette consumption decreased.

Acupuncture Experts Introduce the Treatment

If you have decided to undergo this procedure, consult a skilled and well-trained acupuncturist. Most of these specialists offer a more personalised service and counselling to patients. Sometimes, they use herbal supplements to help your efforts in smoking cessation even more effective.

As mentioned earlier, during the application of the procedure, filiform needles will be placed in certain acupoints on the ear cartilage, on the hands and wrists. Normally, thirty minutes is the allotted duration for the treatment. An acupuncturist may use the combination of wrists and ear placements as well as utilising electric current at a mild level to promote the effect of the needle within the patient's body.

Compared to many other nicotine replacement products and medication, acupuncture has no side effects. This is because the procedure does not utilise substances that are chemically manufactured. Also, during therapy do not worry about gaining weight because this method can also help patients reduce their food cravings and curb their appetite.

Thus, if you are sick and tired of these medications and therapies in smoking cessation, maybe it is about time you consider this holistic form of healthcare. Just make sure that you look for a skilled acupuncturist. Before long you will be able to liberate yourself from smoking, you just have to do your part, be committed, and you will be able to stop completely.

Acupuncture Can Help Patients with Migraines

In a comparative study on conventional medical care, it was discovered that acupuncture could help patients suffering from migraines. Acupuncture can also prevent migraine occurrences in some cases, which helps patients to enjoy a better quality life.

In understanding the manner of how this method can aid people with migraines, you have to be aware of its principle, which hails from the ancient Chinese medicine that believes in the imbalance of the blood and energy flow, which is the root cause of this ailment.

To treat the patient, the specialist will insert hair-like needles into certain areas of the body to improve the flow of the blood in the brain, which will result in relief for the patient; pain will be reduced with migraines happen again.

Through the needles, the serotonin levels will be balanced which will affect the flow of the blood vessels. Serotonin levels are also known as neurotransmitters, which have a key role in migraine attacks. When the patient attends their sessions frequently, they will experience more improvements, even coming to a stage where certain contact points are no longer necessary.

It is amazing to discover the end result of the procedure, which may cut down the fifteen to twenty days of agonising pain to eight days. In addition to that, you will be liberating yourself from taking as much medication as before.

Acupuncture can treat migraines, allowing for people to return to their daily lives. This means no more missing work, school or any other commitments.

Nevertheless, the result of the treatment of acupuncture for one patient may be different for another, since the procedure actually depends on the patient and the condition of the attacks he or she experiences. Better yet, there are no side effects when you undergo the procedure, especially if skilful and professional therapists carry it out. They will take care of you so that you don't suffer from pneumothorax and hematoma. Ensure that they sterilise the needles they use or use disposal needles for every client in order to prevent contact with dangerous communicable diseases like hepatitis or HIV.

For more than two decades, people in the United States have opted to practice this alternative form of healthcare. However, there is a need to perform more studies to discover other areas where acupuncture can be very useful aside from treating certain addictions and severe conditions.

Also, more tests needs to be conducted to prove that acupuncture can aid people with migraines, although there is one test that has proven it is true. If you are in doubt, you can continue to rely on conventional medications prescribed by your doctor until such time that you will obtain a published result, but if you cannot wait and decide to give acupuncture a try, you may come across something that works much better for you.

You can ask your doctor for a list of skilled practitioners they can refer, since some medical practitioners have accepted the alternative forms of medicine which can be good to patients. You can also look for acupuncturists online, just ensure that they are recognised and certified by the National

Certification Commission for Acupuncture and Oriental Medicine.

In addition, try to introduce changes to your lifestyle that can trigger factors for migraine attacks. Number one on the list is stress, so give yourself enough exercise and rest, as well as maintaining a balanced diet.

Moreover, it is good if your HMO covers acupuncture procedures. Today, some insurance providers and HMO's cover if not all, some of the costs of acupuncture, however they are often subject to some restrictions.

Acupuncture and Autism

According to a number of studies, the number of children diagnosed with autism has increased. Until today, medical practitioners had not yet discovered how to treat this illness, which is one reason why some patients explore alternative forms of treatment, one of them being acupuncture.

Acupuncture is a form of holistic healthcare which is used in preventing and treating particular diseases. The main tool used in performing this procedure is very small needles which are inserted to the acupoints of the patient's body.

Autism is a long-term disorder in the brain, which is characterised by deficiency in social communication, language and cognition. Children who are diagnosed as autistic may also encounter secondary problems like irritability, aggression, stereotypes, negativism, hyperactivity, temper tantrums, volatile emotions, obsessive-compulsive behaviours and short attention spans.

In some preliminary studies, it was revealed that symptomatic relief for children affected by autism, through acupuncture. At first, the procedure may not be easy, but it is believed to help in the long run. While conventional therapy requires a child to remain still, acupuncture treatment does not. Patients will only experience slight quick pricks on their bodies' vital points.

To understand how effective acupuncture is to children, a test was conducted in the US. Twenty two respondents participated and were given one treatment every other day within the period of four months. After the test treatment, twenty out of twenty-two children experienced impressive improvements. In fact, two of these respondents have cerebral blood flow, however, before and after the treatment the blood flow between the right and left cerebrum showed no changes.

Other than traditional acupuncture, tongue acupuncture was explored as well as in helping children with autism. In a preliminary study in Hong Kong, the results showed that majority of the thirty respondents showed functional changes on various levels which depended on the severity of the disability and age of the patient. After the TAC sessions, functional improvements were noticed particularly for poor balance in walking, spasticity (tiptoeing or scissoring), drooling and ataxia. It was found that after one or two TAC courses, functional improvements were developed. TAC was well-tolerated by most children, since it only produced minor bleeding and occasional pain.

Tongue acupuncture was explored in some studies because there is a relation between the heart and the tongue through the meridians that branches out to all the organs of the body. According to the principles of this method, the tongue can induce the condition of other organs in the body, which is why the method can provide relief to a person suffering from autism.

Some do not believe that acupuncture can single-handedly help people suffering from this illness, so they combine it with other approaches such as attending communication schools and following a particular diet to help develop the mood of the patient.

Until a cure is found, one can opt for this alternative method that may produce improvements, even in a short period of time. Only time can tell when a cure will be discovered, there is much research to still be conducted in order to understand neurological disabilities further. Perhaps an interdisciplinary approach can be utilised by doctors knowing the fact that acupuncture produces positive improvements for children with autism.

Is Acupuncture Helpful to Pregnant Women?

The practice of acupuncture hails back thousands of years ago from ancient Chinese medicine. Recently, this practice was accepted by the Western world, particularly in the United States. It has been discovered that acupuncture can be an effective method if assistance is needed with fertility. Acupuncture focuses on the flow of energy, and can help with one's Qi. Acupuncture can be very helpful with fertility problems, and many men and women have decided to give it a try.

In today's society, there are many older women who are trying to conceive and have a child. Sometimes, this can prove difficult because of fertility problems. There are many practices including acupuncture that may prove effective in treating these problems. In most cases, acupuncture is prescribed to women who have hormone imbalance or blockage of the fallopian tubes. Acupuncture may go together with TCM methods, which are effective remedies against infertility in women. Men can also achieve great benefits from this alternative form of healthcare. According to sources, acupuncture can help treat male infertility due to low sperm count. Apparently, this remedy is extremely popular. In some cases, kidney energies are treated, and herbal supplements are taken, while patients undergo acupuncture sessions

Patients who undergo acupuncture may experience little negative effects within their whole body. This is one reason why the person's body reacts to the effects of infertility problems. Acupuncture does not cure the symptoms of an illness in the body; instead it will determine the main cause of the problem and treat it. In general, acupuncture is used in order for the patient to achieve a healthier wellbeing. It does not really cure infertility but allows you to have a less stressed lifestyle, and at the same time allows traditional treatments on infertility to work better. Through you may choose to conceive through artificial insemination or through other conceiving methods, acupuncture may still help, it will help your body get to a good place of energy balance.

Once the infertility problems of the couple have been dealt with and the woman successfully conceives, some types of acupuncture can still be useful after conception. The practice of acupuncture can help women attain relief from certain cravings and pain. It will also create a healthier environment for the fetus. Subsequent to the delivery of the baby, the mother's energy will be consumed, thus it would be better for her to go back to the acupuncturist again and undergo another session to regain her energy which she use in battling against a variety of negative feelings and postpartum depressions.

Although acupuncture is not prescribed to everyone, it can be utilised as a tool for both husband and wife all throughout the pregnancy period, prior to pregnancy and after. According to studies that carefully research this type of treatment, a large success rate was found. If you are having infertility problems, it might be worth your time to consult your doctor to see if acupuncture may be a good option for you.

Can Acupuncture Treat Fibromyalgia?

Fibromyalgia is an illness that has an effect on numerous individuals, and as of today, has no cure. Nevertheless, there are some treatments that a patient can opt for to relieve pain temporarily. Individuals with fibromyalgia experience pain in their muscles, as well as in their joints, causing more problems like trouble sleeping, stiffness, and fatigue. As patients continue to look for alternative methods of treatment, some will choose acupuncture, which is believed to be one of the most effective alternative treatment techniques. Indeed, most patients find success in treating this illness through acupuncture, as well as other traditional practices. If you have friends or relatives who suffer fibromyalgia, you can suggest that they undergo acupuncture, which may somehow relieve the symptoms of this illness.

Due to the minimal side effects of acupuncture, most people choose this procedure. Patients gladly report that they experience slight relief after leaving the doctor's clinic compared to the twinges they feel upon arriving. During the procedure, acupuncturists typically use needles, which are as thin as hair. They will insert these needles to stimulate the body of the patient. Some patients feel a delicate pinch when the needles are inserted. Nevertheless, if the insertion is done properly, acupuncture will be performed safely and most patients will feel no pain. Therefore, it is wise to look for a professional therapist.

Patients should have regular treatment to help with the symptoms of fibromyalgia. Most acupuncturists use needles, however, some utilise warming and cupping techniques to get rid of the energies that cause pains to the joints. The procedure is performed within a short period of time. Afterwards, patients will achieve instant relief from the pain in their muscles. However, there are some patients who do not experience relief in any way. Thus, it is important to consult your therapist first to determine if acupuncture would be ideal for your needs, aside from the fact that you will be spending a large amount of money when you go through the process. According to most patients, to achieve best results, they suggest going for repeat sessions of acupuncture. Therefore, plan ahead and be wise in spending, as this could be another expense on your part, which will need to be included in your budget every week.

We cannot deny the fact that in some way or another, this alternative treatment can help patients with fibromyalgia, although there is only a little evidence on this fact compared to the testimonies of the patients who tried acupuncture. At some point, studies should be carried out to further determine if acupuncture is effective for treating this disease.

Many people suffering from fibromyalgia have already experienced effective results through the practice of acupuncture. Before you seek out an acupuncturist, consult your regular physician to find out if acupuncture can work well with your condition. If they believe it is the right course of action for you they can assist in finding an acupuncturist that can help you.

Factors to Consider When Looking for an Acupuncture School

The practice of acupuncture started to flourish in the US in 1982. Presently, there are fifty schools offering trainings for this type of treatment and three thousand licensed acupuncturists practicing in the country. If you want to join in this practice, here are some ideas that could help you in looking for a good acupuncture school.

As mentioned, there are fifty schools in the country, which are all recognised by the National Commission for Acupuncture and Oriental Medicine. These schools are also accredited by the Department of Education, as some of them offer master's degrees.

You can also search about these schools online, try to contact them and ask questions about the school, the tuition fee cost, student teacher ratio, consultation services to students and alumni and whether they have a well-equipped library that contains sufficient resources on ancient Chinese medicine.

If you can find a school near your community, you should consider this as a good option, this way you don't have to worry about the added cost of board and lodging. Studying this alternative method of medicine is a long-term investment, if you cannot afford the tuition fee of the school you want to go to, ask if they offer scholarships or if they have aid programme grants. Or you can also inquire about scholarship grants from the federal government, usually offered to with the federal government for scholarship grants, which they usually award to deserving students, who desires to study in a school recognised by the National Commission for Acupuncture and Oriental Medicine.

After you graduate, you have to prepare yourself for taking the state board exam on acupuncture practice, since this is a necessary requirement. However, there are some states in the country that do not require this.

During your educational training you will study massage and body therapy, anatomy, and other sciences. You will be learning all of the theories of the practice before reaching third year, once you reach the third year level you put them into practice through trainings. Meanwhile, some schools offer a five-year programme on acupuncture practice, whereas, others allow you to finish a three-year programme.

Many schools of acupuncture now offer online programmes for students who are not able to physically attend classes because of distances or other outside circumstances. This is another option you may wish to consider.

If you opt for a distance programme online, you can choose to study when the timing is right for you. The program covers theory, history and techniques of acupuncture. Tools for the improvement of clinical expertise include acupuncture videos and DVDs, which are perfect for students and acupuncturists.

Most graduates of the study of acupuncture start their own practice, while others are employed in clinics or work with other professionals who are chiropractors, naturopaths or other specialists who are also concentrating on Oriental Medicine.

On average, an acupuncturist earns approximately $45,000 annually; however it may increase as they gain more experience or have more years of practice under their belt. If you work hard and become a specialist in the field of acupuncture you can earn a very high salary. You just have to ensure you perform each treatment properly because one error can cause you to lose everything you've worked so hard for.

Degrees in the Study of Acupuncture

Before beginning a career in acupuncture you need both a degree and a licence in order to practice. This is not difficult to attain, you can get your degree in three years in an accredited school. These accredited schools train students to perform numerous techniques related to acupuncture. This includes treating ailments, which result from occupational stress, allergies, emphysema, arthritis, gastrointestinal stress, depression, headaches, hypertension and many more.

Through hands on application and demonstration discussion, students will learn the practice after enrolling in such courses. Other basic courses in traditional medicine that are made part of the curriculum are biosciences, anatomy, herbal medicine, medical terminology, acupressure and moxibustion. Some schools require students to study nutrition and several forms of research.

After a student obtains a degree in acupuncture, they will start to earn from on entry level position taking home $40,000 or more a year. As their years of experience add up, that salary can often double or triple.

For those searching for good school that offers a degree in acupuncture, it may be best to look online and determine which offers the best programme, and which school is suitable for your needs.

At present, it is not any more difficult to look for a training school, as the number of institutions that offer degrees in acupuncture have increased since 1982 upon the establishment of the Council of Colleges of Acupuncture and Oriental Medicine (CCAOM) and the Accreditation Commission for acupuncture and Oriental Medicine (ACAOM).

Today, there are about 50 colleges in the country and a few of them even offer master's degree in Acupuncture and Oriental Medicine. So, do not waste your time, start a long-term investment in the study of acupuncture. It does not matter if you are working now or still in high school, because a change in your career may allow you to realise your true calling.

If you want to start now, it would be best to talk with a practitioner about what you need to prepare in order to become an acupuncturist. If you haven't found a training school yet, talk with other students about the curriculum in order to gain an idea of the value of the money and the effort you will be spending, should you pursue the study.

For those who want to practice after graduating, you can work on your own in New York, California, Hawaii, Texas, and Oregon. In some states acupuncture is not yet legal, while there are eight states in country, which have a pending legislation to allow this practice.

As mentioned earlier, the school where you will obtain your degree should be certified by the Council of Colleges of Acupuncture and Oriental Medicine (CCAOM). You should also get a licence by passing a state exam with the exception for those living in the state of California. They have their own board certification exam and regulating body for those who want to practice this profession.

With a degree in acupuncture, you are just a few steps away from becoming your own boss. To master this field, you have to study hard and learn everything you can about the practice.

While more and more people start to accept the practice of acupuncture, you have to remember studying this method is not a replacement to traditional medicine. This is because there are some restrictions as to what you can offer patients. Acupuncture is merely a holistic form of healthcare that can be used as a supplement to science in order to help patients deal with or treat their illnesses.